Juicing recipes for weight loss

A Beginner's Guide to Balancing

Sweetness, Tartness, and Earthiness

in Your Juices

By

Janet Ryles

Table of contents

Introduction

Are you seriously looking for Juicing recipes for weight loss? Here are some Nature's Candy: Strategic Use of Fruits for Weight Loss. In the pursuit of a healthier and more vibrant lifestyle, the role of nutrition stands as a cornerstone. As individuals embark on their wellness journey, the concept of juicing has emerged not merely as a trend but as a potent ally in achieving and sustaining weight loss goals. This book, "Harmony in a Glass: Juicing Recipes for Weight Loss," is crafted with a blend of culinary expertise and nutritional insight to guide readers through a transformative experience.

In these pages, we delve into the artistry of juicing, exploring meticulously curated recipes designed to not only tantalize taste buds but to strategically support weight loss objectives. Backed by the latest nutritional research, each concoction is a symphony of flavors, nutrients, and the promise of a healthier you.

From invigorating green elixirs to antioxidant-rich fruit medleys, "Harmony in a Glass" offers a diverse array of juicing recipes tailored to meet the unique needs of those on the path to weight management. Beyond the refreshing sips, this book aims to impart a deeper understanding of the nutritional dynamics at play, empowering readers to make informed choices for sustained well-being.

Whether you are a seasoned juicing enthusiast or a novice eager to explore the benefits of liquid nutrition, this guide provides a roadmap to integrate the power of fresh, vibrant juices into your daily routine. Embrace the synergy of flavors and nutrients as we embark together on a journey towards a healthier, more balanced life.

Let the pages of "Harmony in a Glass" be your companion in discovering the exquisite fusion of taste and wellness that awaits within every juiced drop. Cheers to a healthier, happier you!

Chapter One

Introduction to Juicing for Weight Loss Understanding the Role of Juicing in a Weight Loss Journey

In the opening chapter of "Harmony in a Glass: Juicing Recipes for Weight Loss," we embark on a journey to unravel the foundations of juicing as a powerful tool in the pursuit of weight management. We delve into the profound connection between fresh, nutrient-dense juices and their impact on our overall well-being.

Section 1: The Juicing Paradigm

Here, we set the stage by exploring the fundamental principles that underpin the juicing paradigm. Readers gain insights into how juicing goes beyond a mere trend, evolving into a lifestyle choice that can complement and enhance weight loss efforts. We discuss the historical roots of juicing, from ancient practices to its modern resurgence, highlighting its relevance in contemporary wellness.

Section 2: Unveiling the Benefits

The chapter unfolds with an exploration of the myriad benefits that juicing brings to the table. From providing a concentrated source of vitamins and minerals to aiding digestion and detoxification, we dissect the science behind the nutritional potency of freshly pressed juices. This section serves as an enlightening guide, revealing how juicing can act as a catalyst for weight loss while nourishing the body at a cellular level.

Section 3: Integrating Juicing into Daily Life Practicality is key. We guide readers through the seamless integration of juicing into daily routines, addressing common challenges and offering tips on creating a sustainable juicing habit. From time management to ingredient selection, this section provides actionable insights, ensuring that juicing becomes a realistic and enjoyable aspect of one's lifestyle.

Section 4: Setting Expectations Realistic expectations are crucial for any wellness journey. We discuss what individuals can anticipate in terms of initial results and long-term benefits. By understanding the gradual nature of weight loss through juicing, readers are empowered to embark on their path with patience and commitment.

Section 5: Cultivating Mindful Eating

Beyond the physical aspects, we explore the mindfulness that accompanies juicing. By fostering a deeper connection to the ingredients and the act of juicing itself, individuals can cultivate a more conscious approach to their overall dietary choices. This mindfulness forms a cornerstone for sustainable weight loss and improved eating habits.

In essence, Chapter 1 lays the groundwork for a holistic exploration of juicing as a dynamic and beneficial component of a weight loss journey. As readers conclude this introductory chapter, they are equipped with a foundational understanding of the transformative potential that awaits within the pages of "Harmony in a Glass."

Chapter Two

Essentials of Juicing Choosing the Right Juicer: A Buyer's Guide

As we delve into Chapter 2 of "Harmony in a Glass: Juicing Recipes for Weight Loss," the focus shifts to the core tools of the trade—juicers. This chapter serves as a comprehensive buyer's guide, providing readers with the essential knowledge to make informed decisions when selecting the ideal juicer for their needs.

Section 1: Types of Juicers

We begin by dissecting the diverse landscape of juicers, from centrifugal to masticating and triturating models. Each type is examined in detail, shedding light on its mechanics, pros, and cons. Readers gain a nuanced understanding of how different juicers extract juice, and the impact these mechanisms have on nutrient retention and juice quality.

Section 2: Features to Consider

Not all juicers are created equal. This section navigates readers through the crucial features to consider when evaluating juicers. From motor power and speed settings to ease of cleaning and noise levels, we empower individuals to prioritize aspects that align with their lifestyle and juicing preferences.

Section 3: Quality of Ingredients

The quality of ingredients is paramount to the success of any juicing endeavor. Here, we guide readers in selecting the freshest and most nutrient-dense produce. Emphasis is placed on sourcing organic options when possible and exploring local markets to maximize the nutritional benefits of each juice.

Section 4: Storage and Preservation

Once the juice is extracted, understanding proper storage and preservation techniques becomes crucial. This section outlines the best practices for maintaining the freshness and nutritional integrity of juices. From choosing suitable containers to optimizing refrigerator storage, readers learn how to make the most of their juicing efforts.

Section 5: Troubleshooting and Maintenance

Even the most reliable juicers may encounter issues over time. This section equips readers with troubleshooting skills, addressing common problems, and providing maintenance tips to extend the lifespan of their juicing equipment. A well-maintained juicer ensures a seamless and consistent juicing experience.

In essence, Chapter 2 serves as a holistic guide, empowering readers with the knowledge required to embark on their juicing journey with confidence. By the chapter's conclusion, individuals will possess the insights needed to choose, use, and maintain a juicer that aligns seamlessly with their lifestyle and wellness goals.

Chapter Three

Nutritional Foundations Exploring Nutrient-Rich Ingredients for Weight Loss

Chapter 3 of "Harmony in a Glass: Juicing Recipes for Weight Loss" is a deep dive into the nutritional foundations that form the backbone of effective weight management through juicing. This chapter equips readers with a profound understanding of the essential nutrients found in various ingredients and their role in promoting overall health and weight loss.

Section 1: The Power of Phytonutrients

We kick off by unraveling the world of phytonutrients—plant compounds responsible for the vibrant colors of fruits and vegetables. Readers learn about the diverse benefits of phytonutrients, from antioxidant properties to anti-inflammatory effects, and how their inclusion in juicing recipes contributes to a robust health profile.

Section 2: Micronutrients for Vitality

Micronutrients, including vitamins and minerals, play a pivotal role in cellular functions and metabolic processes. This section meticulously explores the micronutrient content of commonly juiced ingredients, guiding readers to craft nutrient-rich combinations that support energy metabolism, immune function, and overall vitality.

Section 3: Fiber and Satiety

Fiber is a key player in the weight loss game, promoting satiety and supporting digestive health. We delve into the two types of fiber—soluble and insoluble—and their distinct roles in weight management. Readers gain insights into selecting ingredients that provide the right balance of fiber to enhance feelings of fullness and aid in digestion.

Section 4: Understanding Sugar Content

While natural sugars are inherent in fruits, it's crucial to strike a balance. This section educates readers on discerning between natural and added sugars, and how to make mindful choices to manage sugar intake through juicing. We provide strategies to sweeten juices without compromising nutritional integrity.

Section 5: The Synergy of Nutrient Combinations

Creating harmonious nutrient combinations is an art. Here, we guide readers in pairing ingredients strategically to amplify nutritional benefits. From vitamin C enhancing iron absorption to combining fats for better fat-soluble vitamin absorption, readers learn the science behind nutrient synergy and its application in juicing.

In conclusion, Chapter 3 transforms juicing from a mere extraction process to a nuanced exploration of nutrition. Armed with a profound understanding of the nutritional foundations, readers are poised to craft juices that not only tantalize the taste buds but serve as potent allies in their weight loss journey.

Chapter Four

Building Balanced Flavors Crafting Delicious Combinations for Palate Pleasure

In Chapter 4 of "Harmony in a Glass: Juicing Recipes for Weight Loss," the focus turns to the art of flavor balancing in juicing. This chapter is a sensory exploration, guiding readers through the intricate process of creating juices that are not only nutritionally robust but also delightfully palatable.

Section 1: The Science of Taste

We begin by unraveling the science of taste and exploring the five primary taste sensations—sweet, sour, salty, bitter, and umami. Readers gain insights into how these taste elements interact, laying the foundation for crafting well-rounded and satisfying juice recipes.

Section 2: Balancing Sweetness, Tartness, and Earthiness

Understanding the interplay between sweetness, tartness, and earthy undertones is crucial to creating juices that appeal to a variety of taste preferences. This section provides a detailed exploration of ingredients that contribute to each flavor profile, empowering readers to experiment with diverse combinations.

Section 3: The Role of Aromatics

Aromatics add depth and complexity to juicing recipes. We delve into the world of aromatic ingredients like herbs and spices, discussing how their inclusion can elevate the sensory experience of a juice. Readers learn to balance aromatic notes for a nuanced and satisfying flavor profile.

Section 4: Creative Ingredient Pairings

Juicing is a canvas for creativity. This section inspires readers with inventive ingredient pairings that go beyond the conventional. From unexpected fruit and vegetable combinations to the inclusion of superfoods, readers are encouraged to think outside the box and tailor juices to their tastes.

Section 5: Addressing Taste Preferences and Restrictions

Tastes vary, and dietary restrictions abound. This section offers strategies for tailoring juices to specific taste preferences and accommodating dietary restrictions. Whether catering to a sweet tooth or navigating a low-sugar diet, readers learn how to customize recipes without compromising nutritional benefits.

In essence, Chapter 4 transforms juicing from a nutritional necessity into a sensory experience. By the chapter's conclusion, readers are equipped with the knowledge to create juices that not only support weight loss goals but also gratify the palate, making the juicing journey a delightful and fulfilling one.

Chapter Five

Green Elixirs for Weight Management Kaleidoscope of Greens: Spinach, Kale, and More

Chapter 5 of "Harmony in a Glass: Juicing Recipes for Weight Loss" takes a focused dive into the world of green juices—a potent elixir for weight management. This chapter explores the nutritional richness of green vegetables and how their incorporation into juices can amplify the benefits of weight loss.

Section 1: The Green Advantage

The chapter kicks off by elucidating the unique nutritional advantages that green vegetables bring to the juicing table. Readers gain an understanding of the rich array of vitamins, minerals, and antioxidants found in greens, setting the stage for why they are a cornerstone of weight-conscious juicing.

Section 2: The Stars of the Green Ensemble

Spinach, kale, chard, and other leafy greens take center stage in this section. Each green is examined for its distinct nutritional profile and flavor contributions. Readers are guided on how to harness the benefits of these leafy powerhouses while creating delicious and satisfying green elixirs.

Section 3: Chlorophyll Magic

Chlorophyll, the green pigment in plants, holds remarkable benefits for health. This section explores the role of chlorophyll in detoxification and its potential impact on weight loss. Readers learn how to maximize chlorophyll intake through green juices, promoting cellular health and balance.

Section 4: Balancing Greens with Fruits and Aromatics

While greens offer a nutritional powerhouse, balancing their earthy flavors with sweet fruits and aromatic ingredients is an art. This section provides practical tips on achieving harmonious blends, ensuring that green juices are not only nutritious but also palatably enjoyable.

Section 5: Tailoring Green Juices to Dietary Goals

Recognizing that dietary goals vary, this section addresses how to customize green juices based on specific weight management objectives. Whether the aim is to boost metabolism, enhance digestion, or increase energy levels, readers gain insights into tailoring green elixirs to meet individual needs.

In conclusion, Chapter 5 invites readers to embrace the vibrant world of green juices as a key component of their weight loss journey. By understanding the nutritional nuances of greens and mastering the art of balancing flavors, individuals are empowered to incorporate these kaleidoscopic elixirs into their daily routine for both health and pleasure.

Chapter Six

Fruit Infusions for a Sweet Boost Nature's Candy: Strategic Use of Fruits for Weight Loss

In Chapter 6 of "Harmony in a Glass: Juicing Recipes for Weight Loss," we delve into the delightful realm of fruit-infused juices—a sweet and nutritious avenue for supporting weight loss goals. This chapter explores the vibrant spectrum of fruits, their unique nutritional contributions, and the art of incorporating them into juices for both taste and wellness.

Section 1: The Nutritional Bounty of Fruits

We commence by unraveling the nutritional bounty that fruits bring to the juicing palette. From vitamins and antioxidants to natural sugars and fiber, readers gain a comprehensive understanding of the diverse benefits offered by different fruits, setting the stage for crafting balanced and nutritious fruit-infused juices.

Section 2: Strategic Fruit Selection for Weight Management

Not all fruits are created equal, especially in the context of weight loss. This section provides insights into selecting fruits strategically, emphasizing those with lower sugar content, high fiber, and metabolism-boosting properties. Readers learn to curate fruit combinations that align with their weight management objectives.

Section 3: Harnessing Antioxidant Power

Fruits are rich in antioxidants, which play a crucial role in supporting overall health. We delve into the antioxidant profiles of various fruits, guiding readers to create juices that combat oxidative stress and inflammation, contributing to a holistic approach to weight management.

Section 4: Blending Sweet and Tart Notes

Balancing sweetness with tartness is an essential aspect of crafting satisfying fruit-infused juices. This section explores the synergy between sweet and tart fruits, offering tips on achieving delightful flavor combinations that not only please the palate but also contribute to satiety.

Section 5: Innovative Fruit Pairings and Superfoods

Creativity takes center stage as we explore innovative fruit pairings and the inclusion of superfoods. Readers are inspired to experiment with exotic fruits, herbs, and nutrient-dense additives to elevate the nutritional profile of their juices. This section encourages a playful approach to juicing while maintaining a focus on health-conscious choices.

In essence, Chapter 6 invites readers to savor the natural sweetness of fruits while strategically incorporating them into their weight loss journey. By the chapter's conclusion, individuals are equipped with the knowledge and inspiration to craft fruit-infused juices that not only tantalize the taste buds but also contribute to their overall well-being.

Chapter Seven

Detoxifying Elixirs Lemon-Ginger Zest: A Detoxifying Duo

In Chapter 7 of "Harmony in a Glass: Juicing Recipes for Weight Loss," the focus shifts to detoxification through the exploration of invigorating and cleansing elixirs. This chapter delves into the powerful combination of lemon and ginger, unlocking their potential to aid in detoxifying the body and supporting weight loss.

Section 1: The Detoxification Imperative

We commence by examining the critical role of detoxification in the context of weight loss. Readers gain insights into how the body eliminates toxins and the potential impact of a well-designed detoxifying juice regimen. This section sets the stage for understanding the synergy between lemon and ginger in this detoxification process.

Section 2: Lemon's Citrus Brilliance

Lemon, with its high vitamin C content and alkalizing properties, takes the spotlight in this section. Readers discover how lemon contributes to liver function, digestion, and hydration. Practical tips on selecting and incorporating fresh lemon into juices are provided, ensuring optimal detoxification benefits.

Section 3: The Warming Power of Ginger

Ginger, celebrated for its anti-inflammatory and digestive properties, is explored in detail. Readers learn about the bioactive compounds in ginger that contribute to detoxification and how to harness its unique flavor and warmth in juicing recipes. Tips on preparing and juicing ginger root effectively are shared.

Section 4: Crafting Detoxifying Blends

This section guides readers in crafting effective and flavorful detoxifying blends. Lemon and ginger are paired with complementary ingredients to enhance the detoxification process while creating juices that are both refreshing and invigorating. The chapter includes a variety of recipes suitable for different taste preferences.

Section 5: Detoxification Beyond the Juice

Detoxification is not confined to the glass; lifestyle factors play a crucial role. This section explores practices that support detoxification beyond juicing, such as hydration, exercise, and adequate sleep. Readers gain a holistic understanding of how lifestyle choices synergize with detoxifying elixirs for optimal weight management.

In conclusion, Chapter 7 invites readers to embrace the synergistic power of lemon and ginger in crafting detoxifying elixirs. By understanding the science behind detoxification and incorporating these vibrant ingredients into juicing, individuals are empowered to embark on a cleansing journey that complements their weight loss goals.

Chapter Eight

Juicing as a Meal Replacement Creating Satisfying and Nutrient-Dense Meal Replacement Juices

Chapter 8 of "Harmony in a Glass: Juicing Recipes for Weight Loss" navigates the terrain of meal replacement juices—a strategic approach to nourishing the body while supporting weight control. This chapter explores the principles of crafting satisfying, nutrient-dense juices that can serve as effective and health-conscious meal substitutes.

Section 1: The Concept of Juicing as a Meal Replacement

The chapter begins by elucidating the rationale behind using juices as meal replacements. Readers gain insights into the potential benefits of integrating nutrient-dense juices into meal plans, including calorie control, increased nutrient absorption, and the convenience of a quick and portable meal option.

Section 2: Essential Nutrients for Meal Replacement Juices

Building on the nutritional foundations explored in earlier chapters, this section details the essential nutrients required for creating balanced meal replacement juices. From proteins and healthy fats to a spectrum of vitamins and minerals, readers learn to curate juices that provide a comprehensive array of nutrients necessary for satiety and well-being.

Section 3: Protein-Rich Ingredients for Sustained Energy

Protein is a key component of meal replacement juices for its role in promoting fullness and sustaining energy levels. This section explores plant-based protein sources suitable for juicing, such as nuts, seeds, and certain vegetables. Readers discover how to incorporate these ingredients strategically to enhance the protein content of their meal replacement juices.

Section 4: Balancing Macros for Weight Control

Maintaining a balanced ratio of macronutrients—carbohydrates, proteins, and fats—is crucial for effective weight control. This section guides readers in achieving the right macro balance in their meal replacement juices, ensuring sustained energy, satiety, and optimal nutritional intake.
Section 5: Creating Filling and Flavorful Meal Replacement Juices
Practical tips and recipes are provided in this section to help readers craft meal replacement juices that are both filling and flavorful. From savory options to sweet blends, the chapter encourages experimentation with ingredients and flavors to suit individual preferences.

In essence, Chapter 8 equips readers with the knowledge and tools to leverage juicing as a strategic meal replacement approach in their weight management journey. By understanding the principles of nutrient balance and satiety, individuals can embrace meal replacement juices as a convenient and health-conscious option for achieving and maintaining their weight loss goals.

Chapter Nine

Hydration and Weight Loss The Link Between Proper Hydration and Weight Management

In Chapter 9 of "Harmony in a Glass: Juicing Recipes for Weight Loss," we explore the symbiotic relationship between hydration and weight management. This chapter sheds light on the pivotal role of adequate hydration in supporting overall health and its specific impact on optimizing weight loss efforts through juicing.

Section 1: The Importance of Hydration

The chapter begins by emphasizing the fundamental importance of hydration for the body's optimal functioning. Readers gain insights into how proper hydration influences metabolism, digestion, and the elimination of toxins, laying the groundwork for understanding its critical role in weight management.

Section 2: Hydrating Through Juicing

Juices are not only flavorful; they are also a valuable source of hydration. This section delves into the hydrating properties of various fruits and vegetables commonly used in juicing. Readers learn how to craft juices that not only contribute to hydration but also offer additional nutritional benefits to support weight loss.

Section 3: The Water Content of Ingredients

Different ingredients have varying water content, influencing the overall hydrating effect of juices. This section provides a comprehensive guide to the water content of popular juicing ingredients, empowering readers to tailor their juices based on hydration needs and preferences.

Section 4: Electrolytes and Hydration Balance

Electrolyte balance is a crucial aspect of effective hydration. We explore the role of electrolytes such as potassium and sodium in maintaining fluid balance in the body. Readers gain insights into incorporating electrolyte-rich ingredients into their juices to enhance hydration and support overall well-being.

Section 5: Timing and Hydration Strategies

Timing matters when it comes to hydration. This section discusses strategic timing for consuming hydrating juices throughout the day, optimizing their impact on metabolism and satiety. Practical hydration strategies are shared, ensuring readers can integrate juicing into their daily routine for consistent and effective hydration.

In conclusion, Chapter 9 underscores the intrinsic connection between hydration and weight management, highlighting how juicing can be a delicious and hydrating tool in this endeavor. By understanding the principles of hydration and incorporating them into juicing practices, individuals can elevate their weight loss journey while fostering overall health and well-being.

Chapter Ten

Juicing Challenges and Solutions Overcoming Common Juicing Hurdles

Chapter 10 of "Harmony in a Glass: Juicing Recipes for Weight Loss" addresses the practical challenges that individuals may encounter on their juicing journey and offers effective solutions to ensure a seamless and rewarding experience.

Section 1: Time Constraints and Convenience
One of the most common challenges is the perception that juicing requires significant time and effort. This section provides time-saving tips, batch juicing strategies, and

insights into streamlining the juicing process without compromising on nutritional quality. Readers learn how to integrate juicing into busy lifestyles for sustained success.

Section 2: Cost Considerations

The perceived cost of juicing can be a barrier for some. This section explores budget-friendly juicing options, smart ingredient choices, and tips for maximizing the value of each juice. Readers discover how to enjoy the benefits of juicing without breaking the bank.

Section 3: Picky Eaters and Flavor Preferences

Addressing the diverse palate preferences of individuals is essential for sustaining a juicing habit. This section provides creative solutions for accommodating picky eaters, experimenting with flavor profiles, and tailoring juices to suit individual tastes. Readers gain insights into making juicing a pleasurable and personalized experience.

Section 4: Nutrient Loss and Pulp Utilization

Concerns about nutrient loss during juicing and the disposal of pulp are common. This section educates readers on minimizing nutrient loss through proper juicing techniques and explores inventive ways to utilize leftover pulp, reducing waste and maximizing nutritional benefits.

Section 5: Storage and Freshness Challenges

Maintaining the freshness of juices and managing storage can be a hurdle. This section offers guidance on proper storage techniques, the use of airtight containers, and tips for preserving the nutritional integrity of juices over time. Readers learn how to overcome freshness challenges for a consistent juicing routine.

In essence, Chapter 10 empowers readers to navigate and conquer common challenges associated with juicing. By providing practical solutions and addressing potential hurdles, individuals are equipped to overcome barriers, ensuring a sustainable and enjoyable juicing practice that aligns with their weight loss goals and lifestyle.

Chapter Eleven

Incorporating Exercise with Juicing Synergizing Physical Activity and Juicing for Optimal Results

Chapter 11 of "Harmony in a Glass: Juicing Recipes for Weight Loss" explores the synergistic relationship between juicing and exercise, illuminating how these two elements can complement each other for enhanced well-being and optimal weight management.

Section 1: Understanding the Exercise-Juicing Connection

This section introduces readers to the fundamental connection between exercise and juicing. The chapter establishes the premise that combining the benefits of regular physical activity with nutrient-rich juices can create a powerful synergy, fostering overall health and supporting weight loss goals.

Section 2: Pre-Workout Juices for Energy and Stamina

Juices can serve as potent pre-workout fuel, providing the body with essential nutrients and hydration. Readers gain insights into crafting juices that offer sustained energy, improved stamina, and enhanced focus, preparing the body for effective and enjoyable exercise sessions.

Section 3: Post-Workout Juices for Recovery and Nourishment

The post-workout period is critical for recovery and replenishment. This section explores the role of juices in post-exercise nutrition, emphasizing ingredients that aid in muscle recovery, hydration, and replenishment of electrolytes. Readers learn to create juices that support the body's recovery process.

Section 4: Hydration Strategies During Exercise

Maintaining proper hydration during exercise is paramount. This section provides practical strategies for incorporating hydrating juices into workout routines, ensuring that individuals stay adequately fueled and hydrated during physical activity. Tips on choosing ingredients that enhance hydration are included.

Section 5: Tailoring Juicing to Exercise Goals

Different forms of exercise have unique nutritional requirements. This section guides readers in tailoring their juicing practices to align with specific exercise goals, whether it's endurance training, strength building, or flexibility exercises. The chapter empowers individuals to customize their juicing routine to enhance their fitness journey.

In conclusion, Chapter 11 encourages readers to view juicing and exercise as complementary components of a holistic approach to health and weight management.

By understanding the nuanced relationship between the two and implementing practical strategies, individuals can unlock the full potential of combining exercise with juicing for optimal well-being.

Chapter Twelve

Maintaining Long-Term Success Strategies for Sustainable Weight Loss Through Juicing

Chapter 12 of "Harmony in a Glass: Juicing Recipes for Weight Loss" delves into the crucial aspects of sustaining success in weight management through juicing. This chapter provides readers with practical strategies, lifestyle considerations, and motivational insights for a sustainable and enduring wellness journey.

Section 1: Establishing Habits for Long-Term Success

The chapter begins by emphasizing the importance of cultivating habits that support long-term success. Readers learn about the power of consistency, gradual changes, and the establishment of sustainable routines to maintain the benefits of juicing for weight loss over time.

Section 2: Creating a Personalized Juicing Routine

Personalization is key to sustaining any lifestyle change. This section guides readers in creating a personalized juicing routine that aligns with their preferences, schedules, and nutritional needs. Practical tips on adapting juicing to individual lifestyles ensure that it becomes an integrated and enjoyable aspect of daily life.

Section 3: Monitoring Progress and Adjusting Goals

Regular monitoring of progress and the flexibility to adjust goals are essential for sustained success. This section discusses effective ways to track changes, celebrate achievements, and reassess goals as needed. Readers gain insights into staying motivated and adapting their approach as they progress on their weight loss journey.

Section 4: Integrating Whole Foods into the Diet

While juicing offers a concentrated source of nutrients, whole foods play a vital role in a balanced diet. This section explores the integration of whole foods alongside juicing, ensuring that individuals receive a comprehensive array of nutrients from a variety of sources for overall health and well-being.

Section 5: Cultivating Mindful Eating Habits

Mindful eating goes beyond the act of juicing; it extends to all aspects of dietary choices. This section encourages readers to cultivate mindful eating habits, foster a deeper connection to food, appreciate flavors, and make conscious choices that support their weight loss goals.

Section 6: Emotional Well-Being and Weight Management

Addressing the emotional aspects of eating is crucial for sustained success. This section explores the connection between emotions and eating habits, providing strategies for managing stress, emotional eating, and maintaining a positive mindset throughout the weight loss journey.

In essence, Chapter 12 serves as a guidepost for readers embarking on a lifelong journey of wellness through juicing. By instilling habits, personalizing routines, and addressing the holistic aspects of well-being, individuals are empowered to navigate the challenges and triumphs of their weight management adventure with resilience and enduring success.

Chapter Thirteen

Recipes for Special Occasions
Juicing for Celebrations and Social Gatherings

Chapter 13 of "Harmony in a Glass: Juicing Recipes for Weight Loss" introduces a delightful exploration into the world of special occasion juicing. This chapter is designed to inspire readers with creative and celebratory juice recipes suitable for various events and social gatherings.

Section 1: The Joy of Juicing for Special Moments

The chapter begins by emphasizing the role of juicing in enhancing special occasions.

Readers gain an understanding of how juicing can contribute to a celebratory atmosphere, providing a healthy and vibrant alternative to traditional beverages during gatherings.

Section 2: Festive and Flavorful Juice Recipes

This section unveils a collection of festive juice recipes crafted for specific occasions. From holiday gatherings to birthdays and festive seasons, readers discover creative combinations that not only cater to the theme of the celebration but also prioritize nutritional value. Recipes include refreshing mocktails, vibrant spritzers, and flavorful punch bowls.

Section 3: Mocktails for Social Elegance

Mocktails, or non-alcoholic cocktails, take center stage in this section. Readers explore recipes that mimic the sophistication and elegance of traditional cocktails while offering a healthier alternative. These mocktails are designed to elevate social occasions without compromising on flavor or nutritional benefits.

Section 4: Interactive Juicing Stations

For interactive and engaging gatherings, this section introduces the concept of juicing stations. Readers learn how to set up interactive juice bars at events, allowing guests to customize their refreshing concoctions. This adds a dynamic and participatory element to social occasions.

Section 5: Incorporating Superfoods and Garnishes

To add a nutritional boost and aesthetic appeal, this section explores the incorporation of superfoods and garnishes into celebratory juices. From chia seeds and acai berries to fresh herbs and edible flowers, readers gain insights into elevating the visual and nutritional allure of special occasion juices.

Section 6: Creating Healthy Toasts

Toasting to special moments can be done with health-conscious alternatives. This section provides recipes for celebratory toasts using nutrient-rich juices. Whether it's a New Year's Eve toast or a wedding celebration, readers discover unique and flavorful ways to raise a glass to joyous occasions.

In conclusion, Chapter 13 encourages readers to embrace the joy of juicing during special occasions. By providing a repertoire of creative and celebratory juice recipes, individuals can enhance the festive atmosphere while promoting health and well-being among friends and loved ones.

Chapter Fourteen

Juicing for Families and Children Nurturing Healthy Habits from an Early Age

Chapter 14 of "Harmony in a Glass: Juicing Recipes for Weight Loss" focuses on the integration of juicing into family life, emphasizing the benefits of cultivating healthy habits for both adults and children. This chapter provides practical insights, recipes, and tips for making juicing an enjoyable and nutritious family activity.

Section 1: The Family Wellness Connection

The chapter begins by highlighting the importance of family wellness and how juicing can be a bonding activity that nurtures healthy habits. Readers gain an understanding of the positive impact that involving the entire family in juicing can have on overall well-being.

Section 2: Kid-Friendly Juicing Basics

Juicing with children requires a tailored approach. This section explores the basics of making juices appealing to kids, from choosing colorful ingredients to incorporating familiar flavors. Readers learn strategies for introducing juicing to children positively and enjoyably.

Section 3: Nutrient-Rich Recipes for Young Palates

A collection of nutrient-rich recipes designed specifically for children takes center stage in this section. These recipes focus on flavors and textures that appeal to young palates while providing essential vitamins and minerals. From fruity concoctions to vibrant vegetable blends, readers discover creative ways to make juicing enticing for children.

Section 4: Family-Friendly Juicing Activities

Creating a positive juicing experience for the whole family involves interactive activities. This section introduces family-friendly juicing games, challenges, and collaborative efforts that turn juicing into an engaging and enjoyable group activity. These activities foster a sense of togetherness and shared health goals.

Section 5: Addressing Concerns and Preferences

Children may have specific preferences and concerns when it comes to juicing. This section addresses common challenges, such as taste preferences, and provides practical solutions for accommodating individual needs within the family. Tips on addressing picky eaters and fostering a positive attitude toward nutritious choices are shared.

Section 6: Education and Empowerment

Empowering children with knowledge about the benefits of juicing forms the core of this section. Readers gain insights into age-appropriate ways to educate children about the nutritional value of different ingredients and the positive impact of making healthy choices. This empowerment fosters a lifelong appreciation for wellness.

In essence, Chapter 14 encourages readers to embrace juicing as a family-oriented and health-promoting activity. By providing practical strategies, recipes, and insights, this chapter empowers families to make juicing an integral part of their shared wellness journey, promoting healthy habits that can last a lifetime.

Conclusion Chapter

Savoring the Journey to Wellness

As we reach the culmination of "Harmony in a Glass: Juicing Recipes for Weight Loss," the journey embarked upon is not just about extracting juices but about crafting a lifestyle that harmonizes nutrition, taste, and well-being. This conclusion reflects on the key takeaways and the profound impact of integrating juicing into a holistic approach to weight management.

Reflecting on the Juicing Odyssey

The conclusion begins by inviting readers to reflect on the odyssey of juicing, emphasizing that it's not merely a dietary choice but a transformative journey. It encourages readers to acknowledge the knowledge gained, the flavors savored, and the positive changes experienced along the way.

Empowerment Through Knowledge

Throughout the book, the emphasis has been on empowerment through knowledge. The conclusion underscores how understanding the science behind juicing, from nutrient profiles to flavor balancing, empowers individuals to make informed choices that resonate with their unique preferences and wellness goals.

The Versatility of Juicing

The versatility of juicing is celebrated in the conclusion. From weight loss to special occasions and family gatherings, juicing has been presented as a flexible and enjoyable practice that adapts to various aspects of life. The conclusion encourages readers to continue exploring the diverse applications of juicing in their daily lives.

Cultivating Sustainable Habits

Sustainability takes center stage in the conclusion. It encourages readers to view juicing not as a temporary fix but as a sustainable habit woven into the fabric of daily routines. The conclusion guides maintaining consistency, adjusting goals, and navigating challenges for enduring success.

Fostering a Culture of Wellness

Ultimately, the book concludes by highlighting that juicing extends beyond the glass—it fosters a culture of wellness. From family bonding to celebratory toasts, juicing becomes a symbol of prioritizing health and savoring life's moments with vibrancy and vitality.

Gratitude for the Juicing Community

The conclusion expresses gratitude to the readers, acknowledging their commitment to exploring the world of juicing for weight loss. It recognizes the diversity of journeys undertaken and the collective effort to foster a community dedicated to well-being.

In essence, the conclusion serves as a heartfelt farewell to the pages of "Harmony in a Glass." It invites readers to continue their

juicing journey with a sense of
empowerment, mindfulness, and a
celebration of the harmonious balance
achieved through the art and science of
juicing.